Fix Your Gut, Fix Your Life

A Practical Reset for Digestion, Energy & Wellness

My Gut Healing Journey: How I Found Relief and You Can Too

✦✦✦

By Shweta Jaiswal

Contents

Acknowledgement

From Constipation to Clarity

This isn't just a book — it's a piece of my healing journey. I was tired of feeling stuck. Constipation, random bloating, fatigue, frustration — it was affecting my focus, my energy, and my life. I wanted answers, but I didn't want complicated science — I wanted clarity.

That's what this guide is for.

If you're someone struggling with gut issues, know this: **You're not lazy. You're not overthinking. Your gut really affects your mind, mood, and life.**

In this book, I've broken down everything I've learned — in the simplest way — so you can understand, heal, and glow from within.

You deserve to feel light, calm, and in control of your body.

Let’s heal together.

Chapter One

Why Gut Health is the Root of Everything

When I first heard that "your gut is your second brain," I didn't take it seriously. But after struggling with constant bloating, stubborn constipation, and mood swings, I started learning more — and everything changed.

Your gut is not just about digesting food. It's the core of your energy, emotions, and immunity. When it works well, you feel light, focused, and vibrant. When it's upset, your whole system struggles.

Here's what makes gut health so important:

- **Your gut and brain are connected** through something called the gut-brain axis. This means your mood, thoughts, and anxiety are deeply affected by your digestion.
- **70% of your immunity** comes from your gut. If your digestion is weak, your body becomes more prone to illness.

- **Nutrients are absorbed in your intestines.** Even if you're eating healthy, if your gut isn't working right, your body won't benefit.

I used to ignore these signs — thinking fatigue and brain fog were just part of my routine. But deep down, my gut was calling for help.

This chapter is your reminder: don't ignore the signals. Healing begins here.

Next up: Let's simplify how digestion actually works — no science degree needed!

Chapter Two

Understanding Digestion

Let's Make it Simple

- **Step 1:** It All Starts in the Mouth Digestion begins even before you swallow food. When you smell or see something delicious, your brain sends signals to start producing saliva. Saliva has enzymes (like amylase) that begin breaking down carbohydrates.

→ **Tip from me:** Chew slowly. When I started chewing food properly (at least 20–30 times), my digestion improved naturally.

- **Step 2:** Down the Esophagus After chewing, the food travels down a long tube called the esophagus into the stomach. This movement is called peristalsis — a gentle squeezing action.
- **Step 3: Stomach** — The Breakdown Zone Here, powerful stomach acid (HCL) and enzymes work together to break down proteins and kill bad

bacteria. This acid is crucial — but many people with stress or poor diet have low stomach acid!

→ **Sign of low stomach acid?** Bloating after meals, burping, feeling full quickly.

- **Step 4: Small Intestine** — Absorption Hub Once the food is broken down into smaller bits, it moves into the small intestine. Here, the magic happens: nutrients get absorbed into the blood and sent to cells.

The pancreas and liver also send digestive juices and bile to help digest fats, carbs, and proteins.

- **Step 5: Large Intestine** — Waste & Water Whatever isn't absorbed moves into the large intestine. Water is absorbed here, and healthy gut bacteria (your microbiome) ferment the leftover fiber.

This is where poop is formed.

→ If things go wrong here (too dry, too fast, too slow), constipation or diarrhea shows up.

Fun Fact: The gut has over 100 trillion bacteria. Some are friendly (help with digestion, immunity, and mood). Others are harmful. Balance is key.

Gut-Brain Link (again!) If your digestion is slow or painful, it affects your emotions too. A stressed gut sends danger signals to the brain — and vice versa. It's a loop.

That's why healing digestion = calming the mind, too.

This chapter gives you the foundation. In the next one, we'll talk about the biggest enemy of your gut: stress.

Chapter Three

Stress — The Hidden Enemy of Your Gut

When you're stressed, your body isn't just affected mentally. Your gut takes a hit too.

Stress does more than mess with your mood. It can slow down digestion, cause bloating, and even lead to constipation. The more stress you feel, the more you affect your gut's ability to work efficiently.

Here's why:-

Fight or Flight Mode: When you're stressed, your body goes into 'fight or flight' mode. This is a survival mechanism — your body prepares for danger by diverting energy away from less important functions, like digestion.

Stress and the Gut-Brain Axis: We've talked about how your gut and brain are connected. Stress can actually hijack this connection, triggering symptoms like nausea, constipation, diarrhea, and bloating.

Chronic Stress Leads to Chronic Gut Problems: If stress becomes a regular part of your life, it can lead to long-term digestive issues. Low stomach acid, leaky gut, and imbalance in gut bacteria are just some of the effects of constant stress.

- **My Personal Experience:** When I was stressed, I noticed that my digestive problems became worse. After a tough day at work or an argument, I would feel bloated, exhausted, and sometimes, constipated. It took me a while to realize that my stress levels were directly impacting my gut health.

So, what can you do about it?

- **Relaxation is Key** It's not just about "dealing with stress" — it's about finding ways to relax your nervous system. Techniques like deep breathing, yoga, and even taking walks in nature can help calm the gut and mind.

- **Mindful Eating:** When you eat in a stressed state, your body doesn't digest food properly. Slow down, eat with intention, and try to reduce distractions like TV or your phone during meals.
- **Mindset Shift:** Stress management isn't just about removing stressful things. It's also about changing how we react. Can you see stress as a challenge, not a threat? That mindset shift makes a huge difference.

Chapter Four

Foods for Gut Health — What to Eat (and What to Avoid)

What you eat plays a huge role in how your gut feels and functions. It's not just about 'eating healthy' — it's about feeding your gut the right nutrients it needs to thrive.

There are certain foods that help heal your gut, and others that can do more harm than good.

Let's break it down:

Foods That Help Your Gut Health

- **Probiotics:** These are live bacteria that help balance your gut. Foods like yogurt, kefir, sauerkraut, kimchi, and kombucha are packed with probiotics that can boost your gut health.
- **Prebiotics:** These are the foods that nourish good bacteria in your gut. Think onions, garlic, leeks, bananas, and asparagus.
- **Fiber-Rich Foods:** Foods like oats, beans, lentils, fruits, and vegetables help keep things moving in

your digestive system. Fiber promotes healthy bowel movements and prevents constipation.

- **Healthy Fats:** Omega-3 fatty acids (found in fish, walnuts, flaxseeds) can reduce inflammation and promote gut healing.
- **Bone Broth:** Rich in collagen, amino acids, and minerals, bone broth helps heal the gut lining and improve digestion.

My Personal Experience: When I started including more probiotic-rich foods in my diet, I felt my bloating decrease, my energy levels go up, and my digestion improved. I didn't expect it to be an overnight change, but over time, I noticed a huge difference.

Foods to Avoid for Better Gut Health

- **Processed Foods:** Foods high in refined sugars, artificial sweeteners, and preservatives can cause gut inflammation and disrupt your gut microbiome. Cut back on fast food, sugary snacks, and sodas.
- **Dairy (for some people):** Dairy can cause bloating, gas, and diarrhea, especially for those who are lactose intolerant. If dairy doesn't sit well with you, try lactose-free alternatives or plant-based options like almond or oat milk.
- **Gluten (for some people):** Some individuals may have sensitivities to gluten, which can cause bloating, discomfort, and inflammation. Gluten-free grains like quinoa, rice, and oats are great alternatives.

- **Fried and Fatty Foods:** Heavy, greasy meals can slow down digestion and lead to discomfort. If you're struggling with gut issues, limit your intake of fried foods.
- **Caffeine and Alcohol:** Both can irritate your gut lining and cause bloating and discomfort, especially when consumed in excess.

My Personal Experience: When I eliminated processed foods and cut down on sugary snacks, I noticed my energy levels increased and my digestion improved. I also felt less bloated after meals.

Tips for a Gut-Healthy Diet

- **Eat a Variety of Whole Foods:** Aim for a variety of colorful fruits, vegetables, legumes, whole grains, and healthy fats. A diverse diet ensures that your gut gets a range of nutrients to thrive.

- **Drink Plenty of Water:** Water is essential for digestion and helps move food through your system. Aim to drink at least 8 cups a day.
- **Avoid Overeating:** Eating smaller, more frequent meals can reduce the stress on your digestive system.
- **Listen to Your Body:** Pay attention to how your body responds to different foods. If something makes you feel bloated or uncomfortable, avoid it or find a suitable alternative.

Chapter 5

The Role of Hydration in Gut Health

You've probably heard it a million times: "Drink water." But do you know how important hydration is for your gut?

Water is an essential part of digestion. It helps break down food so your body can absorb nutrients. Without enough water, your digestive system can't function properly, leading to issues like constipation, bloating, and discomfort.

Here's why hydration matters so much for your gut:

How Hydration Supports Digestion

- **Lubrication:** Water helps keep food moving smoothly through your digestive tract. Without enough water, your intestines can become sluggish, leading to constipation and bloating.
- **Digestive Enzyme Activation:** Water helps activate the digestive enzymes that break down

food. These enzymes are crucial for nutrient absorption, which is key for your energy and health.

- **Stool Softening:** If you're struggling with constipation, dehydration is often a culprit. When your body doesn't have enough water, your stool becomes harder and more difficult to pass.
- **Gut Lining Protection:** Proper hydration helps maintain the integrity of your gut lining, which is important for preventing leaky gut syndrome and other digestive issues.

How Much Water Do You Need?

The general recommendation is to drink around 8 cups (2 liters) of water a day. But your hydration needs may vary depending on factors like activity level, climate, and overall health.

My Personal Experience: When I started consciously drinking more water, I noticed that my digestion improved, and my bloating decreased. It wasn't just about drinking a lot of water at once — it was about staying consistently hydrated throughout the day.

Tips to Stay Hydrated

- **Drink Water First Thing in the Morning:** Start your day with a glass of water to kickstart your digestive system and prevent dehydration.
- **Carry a Water Bottle:** Keep a water bottle with you at all times to remind yourself to drink regularly.
- **Add Electrolytes for Better Hydration:** If you're dehydrated or need extra hydration, adding a pinch of salt or a few drops of electrolytes to your water can help you retain fluids.

- **Eat Hydrating Foods:** Many fruits and vegetables have high water content, like cucumbers, watermelon, and oranges. These can help keep you hydrated along with your water intake.
- **Don't Wait Until You're Thirsty:** By the time you feel thirsty, you may already be slightly dehydrated. Make it a habit to sip water throughout the day.

Chapter 6

The Power of Mindset in Healing

Gut health isn't just about the food you eat — it's also about how you feel and think. Yes, your mindset plays a crucial role in your healing journey.

We all know stress can take a toll on the body. But did you know that chronic stress and negative emotions can directly affect your gut? It's called the gut-brain axis, and it's a powerful connection that links your mental state to your digestive system.

The Gut-Brain Connection

Your gut and brain are in constant communication. In fact, your gut has more nerve cells than your spinal cord, which is why it's often called your "second brain." This connection means that what happens in your brain (your emotions, stress levels, etc.) can affect your gut — and vice versa.

- **Stress and Digestion:** When you're stressed or anxious, your body produces more cortisol, the stress hormone. High levels of cortisol can slow down digestion, lead to bloating, constipation, and even cause gut inflammation.

- **Emotions and Digestion:** Anxiety, sadness, and frustration can trigger digestive issues. Ever notice that when you're stressed, you can't digest food properly or feel nauseous? That's your gut reacting to your emotional state.

My Personal Experience: During the most stressful times in my life, my gut issues became worse. When I was overwhelmed with school or personal challenges, I could feel the bloating and discomfort kicking in. But when I started practicing stress-reducing techniques, I saw improvements in my digestion. Healing my mind helped heal my gut.

Shifting Your Mindset for Gut Health

Healing your gut isn't just about diet and supplements — it's also about healing your mindset. Here's how:

- **Practice Gratitude:** Focusing on what you're thankful for can reduce stress and promote better digestion. Start each day by writing down 3 things you're grateful for. This simple habit can improve your mood and help your gut.
- **Meditation and Breathing Exercises:** Meditation, deep breathing, and mindfulness can lower stress levels, balance your nervous system, and promote better digestion.
- **Positive Affirmations:** The way you speak to yourself matters. If you constantly say, "My gut is always upset," you reinforce the cycle of discomfort. Replace negative thoughts with positive affirmations, like "My gut is healing" or "I'm nourishing my body with love."

- **Visualization:** Imagine your gut healing. Visualizing your digestive system working smoothly and effortlessly can actually help improve gut function.
- **Stress Management:** Practice stress-reducing activities like yoga, journaling, or walking. Managing stress is key to improving your gut health.

My Personal Experience: After I began practicing deep breathing and gratitude journaling, I felt calmer and more at ease. My digestive issues seemed less overwhelming. The more I nurtured my mind, the more my gut began to respond positively.

Be Kind to Yourself

One of the most important things I learned was to be kind to myself during the healing process. Healing takes time, and it's okay to have setbacks. Celebrate small victories, and trust the process. Your mind and body need patience, love, and care.

Chapter 7

Lifestyle Changes That Support Gut Health

Your gut is influenced by more than just food — your daily habits and lifestyle choices can play a big part in your digestive health. Let's dive into the lifestyle changes that can make a significant difference in your gut health journey.

1. Sleep: The Unsung Hero

Did you know that your gut needs sleep just like the rest of your body? In fact, poor sleep can negatively affect your gut, leading to issues like bloating, constipation, and indigestion.

When you don't get enough rest, your body produces more cortisol (the stress hormone), which can slow down digestion. Plus, sleep deprivation disrupts the balance of gut bacteria, leading to digestive issues.

How to Improve Sleep:

- Aim for 7-9 hours of sleep each night.

- Create a calming bedtime routine (e.g., reading a book, listening to soothing music).
- Avoid caffeine and electronic screens before bed to help your body relax.
- Sleep in a cool, dark room for better quality sleep.

2. Regular Physical Activity

Movement is key for digestion. When you exercise, you're not only boosting your metabolism, but you're also helping your digestive system work more efficiently.

How Exercise Helps Your Gut:

- Physical activity stimulates the muscles in your intestines, helping food move more easily through your digestive tract.
- It increases blood flow to the digestive organs, improving their function.

- Regular exercise can also help reduce stress, which we know is crucial for gut health.

Tips to Get Moving:

- Go for a 30-minute walk each day to help stimulate digestion.
- Try yoga or gentle stretching to relieve bloating and improve gut function.
- Choose exercises you enjoy so that it's easier to stay consistent.

3. Stress Reduction

We've already touched on how stress affects your gut, but it's worth emphasizing again. Chronic stress can disrupt digestion, leading to conditions like irritable bowel syndrome (IBS) or gut inflammation. Managing stress is essential for gut health.

Ways to Manage Stress:

- **Practice mindfulness and meditation**: These techniques help calm the mind and balance the gut-brain connection.
- **Do breathing exercises**: Deep breathing can activate your parasympathetic nervous system (the "rest and digest" system), promoting better digestion.
- **Spend time in nature**: Nature has a calming effect that can lower cortisol levels and reduce stress.

4. Social Connections and Emotional Support

Your gut health can even be influenced by your relationships and emotional support. When we feel supported and connected to others, our stress levels decrease, and our bodies function better.

How Social Connections Benefit Your Gut:

- **Positive social interactions** help lower stress and improve emotional well-being, which is vital for gut health.
- **Talking through your feelings** can ease emotional tension and prevent gut disturbances caused by anxiety or depression.

5. Healthy Meal Timing and Portion Control

Your gut works best when it's not constantly overworked. Consistent, balanced meal timing is crucial for your digestive health.

Meal Timing Tips:

- Eat smaller, more frequent meals instead of large, heavy meals.

- Avoid eating too close to bedtime, as it can interfere with your digestion and sleep quality.
- Try intermittent fasting (if it works for you) to give your digestive system a break between meals.

My Personal Experience:

When I started making these lifestyle changes — getting more sleep, exercising regularly, and reducing stress — I noticed that my digestive system became more predictable. The bloating decreased, and I felt more energized and in control of my body. These small shifts in lifestyle made a huge difference.

Chapter 8

Foods to Avoid for a Healthy Gut

When you're healing your gut, it's just as important to know what not to eat as it is to know what to eat. Some foods can irritate your digestive system, making bloating, constipation, and other issues worse. Let's talk about the foods that might be sabotaging your gut health and why you should avoid them.

1. Processed Foods

Processed foods, like chips, frozen meals, and sugary snacks, often contain unhealthy fats, added sugars, and artificial ingredients. These can throw off your gut microbiome (the balance of good bacteria in your gut) and cause inflammation.

Why to Avoid Them:

- **Sugar** feeds harmful bacteria and yeast in your gut, leading to imbalance.

- **Artificial additives** (like preservatives, artificial sweeteners, and colorings) can irritate your digestive system and may even disrupt the healthy bacteria in your gut.
- **Refined carbs** (like white bread, pasta, and pastries) can spike blood sugar levels, leading to gut inflammation.

What to Do Instead:

- Opt for whole, unprocessed foods like fresh vegetables, fruits, lean proteins, and whole grains.
- Focus on foods that are rich in fiber, healthy fats, and antioxidants to support gut health.

2. Red Meat and Fatty Cuts of Meat

While a small amount of lean meat can be part of a balanced diet, consuming large amounts of red meat or fatty cuts can cause digestive problems. These meats are hard to digest and can slow down gut motility.

Why to Avoid Them:

- **Saturated fats** in fatty meats can lead to inflammation in the gut.
- Eating too much red meat can disrupt the gut microbiome and make it harder for beneficial bacteria to thrive.
- High-fat diets are often linked to conditions like constipation, bloating, and IBS.

What to Do Instead:

- Choose lean protein sources like chicken, turkey, tofu, fish, or legumes.
- Try plant-based meals that are rich in fiber and easy for your gut to process.

3. Dairy (If You're Sensitive)

For many people, dairy can be a major gut irritant. This doesn't mean you need to cut out dairy completely, but if you're sensitive to it, consuming milk, cheese, and yogurt could lead to bloating, gas, and discomfort.

Why to Avoid It (If You're Sensitive):

- **Lactose intolerance** is common and occurs when your body doesn't produce enough of the enzyme lactase to break down lactose, the sugar in dairy.
- Dairy can also contribute to inflammation, especially in people with autoimmune conditions or irritable bowel syndrome (IBS).

What to Do Instead:

- Opt for dairy alternatives like almond milk, coconut yogurt, or lactose-free products.

- Include more plant-based calcium sources like leafy greens, almonds, and fortified plant milks.

4. Sugary Snacks and Sodas

Consuming high amounts of sugar — especially refined sugar found in candy, sodas, and baked goods — can cause havoc on your gut health. Sugar feeds harmful bacteria and yeast, which can lead to bloating, discomfort, and imbalance in the gut microbiome.

Why to Avoid It:

- **High sugar intake** can increase inflammation in the gut and cause digestive upset.
- Sugary foods contribute to overgrowth of harmful bacteria in the intestines.
- **Sodas** and sugary drinks are also loaded with artificial sweeteners that can negatively impact digestion.

What to Do Instead:

- Choose natural sweetness from fruits like berries, apples, and bananas.
- Drink plenty of water or herbal teas to stay hydrated and help digestion.
- Swap sugary snacks with whole foods like nuts, seeds, and dried fruits (in moderation).

5. Legumes (If You Have Sensitivity)

While legumes like beans, lentils, and chickpeas are rich in fiber and protein, they can be tough to digest for some people, leading to bloating and gas. This is especially true if you're not used to eating a lot of fiber.

Why to Avoid (If You're Sensitive):

- **Fiber overload** can cause gas, bloating, and discomfort in people with sensitive digestion.

- Legumes also contain **anti-nutrients** (such as lectins and phytates) that can irritate the gut lining in sensitive individuals.

What to Do Instead:

- Soaking and sprouting legumes before cooking them can reduce their anti-nutrient content and make them easier to digest.
- If legumes still cause discomfort, focus on other sources of fiber, such as vegetables, whole grains, and fruits.

My Personal Experience: When I started cutting back on processed foods and refined sugars, I noticed an immediate improvement in how I felt. My bloating decreased, my energy levels were more stable, and my digestion became smoother. It wasn’t about a restrictive diet, but about making smarter, healing food choices.

Chapter 9

Foods to Include for a Happy Gut

Healing your gut isn't just about avoiding harmful foods — it's also about eating foods that nurture and support your digestion. Including certain foods in your diet can help repair your gut, reduce inflammation, and keep everything running smoothly.

Let's dive into the top foods you should be adding to your daily meals for a healthier, happier gut.

1. Fiber-Rich Vegetables and Fruits

One of the best things you can do for your gut is to eat foods that are rich in fiber. Fiber acts as a prebiotic, feeding the good bacteria in your gut. It helps with digestion, keeps things moving, and prevents constipation.

Best Options:

- **Leafy greens** like spinach, kale, and arugula are packed with fiber and essential vitamins.

- **Cruciferous vegetables** such as broccoli, cauliflower, and Brussels sprouts promote healthy digestion.
- **Fruits** like berries, apples, pears, and bananas are high in fiber and gentle on the stomach.

Why They're Great:

- Fiber supports the growth of healthy bacteria in your gut, improving your overall gut health.
- They're also rich in antioxidants, which help reduce inflammation.

Tip: Aim to fill half of your plate with fiber-rich vegetables at every meal to keep your gut healthy and happy!

2. Fermented Foods for Gut Health

Fermented foods are a goldmine for gut health. They contain probiotics, which are live bacteria that are beneficial for your digestive system. Eating fermented foods helps replenish the good bacteria in your gut, which can improve digestion, reduce bloating, and boost immunity.

Best Options:

- **Yogurt** (preferably unsweetened and with live active cultures).
- **Kefir**, a fermented milk drink that's even richer in probiotics than yogurt.
- **Sauerkraut** and **kimchi**, fermented cabbage that's full of beneficial bacteria.
- **Miso** and **tempeh**, both made from fermented soybeans, are great plant-based options.

Why They're Great:

- Probiotics help balance the gut microbiome and improve digestive function.
- They can also support your immune system and reduce symptoms like bloating and gas.

Tip: Start with small portions to avoid overloading your digestive system. Gradually increase the amount as your gut adjusts.

3. Healthy Fats

Healthy fats are essential for your overall well-being and also play a vital role in gut health. They help reduce inflammation, support the gut lining, and promote the absorption of fat-soluble vitamins like vitamins A, D, E, and K.

Best Options:

- **Avocados**: Rich in healthy monounsaturated fats, avocados are easy to digest and help soothe the gut.

- **Olive oil**: A staple in the Mediterranean diet, olive oil is anti-inflammatory and supports gut health.
- **Nuts and seeds**: Almonds, walnuts, chia seeds, and flaxseeds are packed with omega-3 fatty acids that support digestion.

Why They're Great:

- Healthy fats help heal the gut lining and reduce gut inflammation.
- They can also help you absorb essential nutrients from other foods.

Tip: Incorporate healthy fats into every meal — just be mindful of portion sizes as they are calorie-dense.

4. Bone Broth

Bone broth is a nutrient-dense food that can do wonders for your gut. Made from simmering animal bones (chicken, beef, or fish) with vegetables, herbs, and spices, bone broth is rich in collagen, gelatin, and amino acids, all of which support gut health.

Why It's Great:

- **Collagen** and **gelatin** help repair the gut lining, promoting digestion and reducing inflammation.
- Bone broth is also soothing to the digestive system and can help reduce bloating and discomfort.
- It’s a great source of minerals like calcium, magnesium, and phosphorus, which support overall health.

Tip: Drink a cup of homemade bone broth daily or use it as a base for soups and stews to support your gut.

5. Prebiotic Foods

Prebiotics are the food for probiotics. They help feed the healthy bacteria in your gut, allowing them to thrive.

Including prebiotic foods in your diet helps support a healthy gut microbiome and improves digestion.

Best Options:

- **Garlic**: Contains inulin, a prebiotic fiber that feeds the good bacteria in your gut.
- **Onions**: Like garlic, onions are high in inulin and promote a healthy gut.
- **Bananas**: Unripe bananas are an excellent source of prebiotic fiber.
- **Asparagus**: Packed with fiber and prebiotics that help nourish your gut bacteria.

Why They're Great:

- Prebiotics promote the growth of beneficial bacteria, improving digestion and overall gut health.

- They help reduce symptoms like bloating and constipation by keeping the gut microbiome balanced.

Tip: Try adding a small portion of prebiotic foods to each meal to keep your gut bacteria well-fed and happy.

My Personal Experience: When I started incorporating these gut-friendly foods into my meals, I felt a noticeable difference. My bloating reduced, my energy improved, and I finally felt lighter and more at ease in my body. It wasn't just about avoiding the "bad" foods, but actively choosing the foods that truly nourished and healed my gut.

Chapter 10

Hydration - The Gut's Best Friend

We've all heard the importance of drinking water, but did you know that hydration plays a crucial role in your gut health? Our bodies are made up of about 60% water, and every cell, including those in our digestive system, relies on it for proper functioning. When we're dehydrated, our digestive system struggles, leading to constipation, bloating, and discomfort.

In this chapter, we'll explore how hydration affects your gut and how to stay properly hydrated for better digestion and overall health.

Why Hydration Matters for Gut Health

1. **Improves Digestion**: Water is essential for the breakdown of food and the absorption of nutrients. Without enough water, your body struggles to digest food effectively, leading to discomfort, constipation, and a sluggish digestive system.

2. **Helps Move Waste**: Proper hydration softens stools and helps them move smoothly through your intestines. If you're not drinking enough water, your body may absorb more water from your stools, leaving them dry and hard — leading to constipation.

3. **Balances Gut Bacteria**: Your gut microbiome thrives on hydration. Water helps maintain the balance of good bacteria in your gut, which is crucial for digestion, immunity, and overall gut health.

4. **Prevents Bloating**: Dehydration can lead to bloating, as your body holds onto water in an attempt to stay hydrated. By staying properly hydrated, you help prevent water retention and reduce bloating.

Signs You Might Be Dehydrated

Dehydration doesn't always look like dry mouth or feeling thirsty. Here are some subtle signs that you might not be drinking enough water:

- Constipation or hard stools.
- Dry or flaky skin.
- Dark-colored urine.
- Feeling fatigued or sluggish.
- Headaches or dizziness.

If you're experiencing any of these signs, it might be time to increase your water intake!

How Much Water Should You Drink?

The amount of water you need depends on various factors like your age, activity level, climate, and health status. However, a general rule of thumb is to aim for around **8 cups (64 ounces)** of water per day. Some experts recommend drinking more if you're active or living in a hot climate.

Tip: A simple way to track your hydration is to carry a water bottle with you and sip regularly throughout the day. You don't have to wait until you're thirsty!

Hydration Tips for Gut Health

1. **Start Your Day with Water**: Begin your morning by drinking a glass of water. This kickstarts your digestion and helps hydrate your body after a night's sleep.
2. **Add Electrolytes**: If you're working out or sweating a lot, consider adding a pinch of sea salt or an electrolyte tablet to your water. Electrolytes help maintain fluid balance in your body, improving hydration and gut function.

3. **Infuse Your Water**: If plain water feels boring, try infusing it with fresh fruits, herbs, or vegetables like lemon, cucumber, or mint. Not only does it make the water taste better, but it also adds extra nutrients!
4. **Eat Water-Rich Foods**: Don't forget that foods like fruits and vegetables also contribute to hydration. Watermelon, cucumbers, strawberries, and celery are all hydrating and help maintain proper fluid balance.
5. **Stay Hydrated Throughout the Day**: Make hydration a habit by drinking water consistently throughout the day, not just when you're thirsty.

Herbal Teas for Gut Health

In addition to water, herbal teas can be a soothing and hydrating option for your gut. Certain herbal teas have digestive benefits and can help reduce bloating, soothe inflammation, and promote better digestion.

Best Herbal Teas for Gut Health:

- **Peppermint tea**: Calms the digestive system and reduces bloating.
- **Ginger tea**: Aids digestion and reduces nausea and bloating.
- **Chamomile tea**: Soothes the digestive tract and helps with inflammation.

Drinking a cup of herbal tea after meals can be a relaxing and beneficial habit for your gut health.

My Personal Experience: When I started focusing on hydration, I noticed a huge difference in my digestion. I felt lighter, had more energy, and didn't struggle with constipation as much. It's such a simple yet powerful habit that made a huge impact on my overall well-being.

Chapter 11

The Impact of Stress on Your Gut Health

We all know how stress can affect our mood, energy, and mental health, but did you know that it can also wreak havoc on your gut? The connection between stress and digestion is powerful and often underestimated. If you've ever experienced an upset stomach or digestive issues during a stressful time, you've felt this connection firsthand.

In this chapter, we'll dive into how stress impacts your gut and share tips on how to manage it to promote healing.

How Stress Affects Your Gut

1. **The Gut-Brain Connection**: Your gut and brain are connected through the **gut-brain axis** — a complex system of nerves, hormones, and biochemicals. This means that stress can send signals to your gut, affecting your digestion, gut bacteria, and overall gut function. When you're stressed, your brain releases chemicals that can slow

down or speed up digestion, leading to discomfort, bloating, or even diarrhea.

2. **Stress Increases Inflammation**: Chronic stress increases levels of cortisol, a stress hormone that can lead to **inflammation** in your gut. This inflammation can disrupt the balance of good and bad bacteria, leading to digestive issues, bloating, and even conditions like **irritable bowel syndrome (IBS)**.

3. **Slows Digestion**: When you're stressed, your body enters a "fight or flight" mode, where blood flow is redirected away from the digestive system. This slows down digestion and can lead to issues like constipation, bloating, and difficulty absorbing nutrients.

4. **Imbalances Gut Bacteria**: Chronic stress can cause an imbalance in your gut microbiome — the

community of bacteria and microorganisms living in your gut. A stressed gut is more likely to have an overgrowth of harmful bacteria and less beneficial bacteria, which can negatively impact digestion, immunity, and overall health.

Signs That Stress Is Impacting Your Gut

- **Constipation** or **diarrhea** when stressed.
- Frequent **bloating** or discomfort.
- Feeling **nauseous** during or after stressful situations.
- Craving unhealthy foods, especially sugary or processed snacks.
- Experiencing **brain fog** or difficulty concentrating.

If any of these sound familiar, stress may be a major contributor to your gut issues.

How to Manage Stress for Better Gut Health

1. **Mindful Breathing**: Deep breathing exercises activate the **parasympathetic nervous system**, also known as the "rest and digest" system. By practicing deep breathing (even for just a few minutes a day), you can calm your nervous system and support healthy digestion. Try **diaphragmatic breathing** or **4-7-8 breathing** to relax.

2. **Meditation**: Regular meditation can help lower cortisol levels, reduce anxiety, and promote relaxation. You don't have to meditate for hours — even a few minutes of mindfulness each day can make a significant impact on your gut and stress levels.

3. **Exercise**: Physical activity is one of the best ways to reduce stress. Whether it's yoga, walking, or

dancing, exercise helps release endorphins (the body's "feel-good" hormones) and reduces stress. Plus, it keeps your digestive system moving and supports healthy gut function.

4. **Prioritize Sleep**: Poor sleep contributes to stress and negatively impacts gut health. Aim for 7-9 hours of quality sleep each night. Try establishing a bedtime routine that includes relaxation techniques, like reading, meditation, or taking a warm bath, to help your body unwind before bed.

5. **Journaling**: Writing down your thoughts can help process emotions, reduce mental clutter, and manage stress. Journaling about your gut health journey can also be empowering, allowing you to track your progress, setbacks, and emotions along the way.

6. **Limit Stimulants**: Caffeine, nicotine, and alcohol can increase stress and disrupt gut health. Consider reducing or eliminating these stimulants, especially when you're feeling stressed, and opt for calming herbal teas instead.

Nourish Your Gut with Stress-Reducing Foods

Some foods have been shown to help manage stress and support gut health. Here's a list of **gut-friendly, stress-reducing foods**:

- **Omega-3-rich foods** (like salmon, flaxseeds, and walnuts) help reduce inflammation in the body and support a healthy gut.
- **Probiotic-rich foods** (such as yogurt, kefir, and fermented vegetables) introduce beneficial bacteria into your gut, helping balance your microbiome.

- **Magnesium-rich foods** (like leafy greens, nuts, and seeds) can relax the nervous system and help manage stress.
- **Vitamin C-rich foods** (like oranges, strawberries, and bell peppers) help reduce cortisol levels and combat stress.

My Personal Experience

There was a time when stress ruled my life. My gut was constantly in turmoil — bloating, constipation, and even skin breakouts. But when I started managing stress with simple practices like deep breathing and meditation, I noticed an incredible difference. I began to feel more grounded, my digestion improved, and I even had more energy.

If stress is a major factor in your life, addressing it can truly transform your gut health.

Chapter 12

Daily Habits for a Healthy Gut Reset

In this final chapter, we'll explore simple, everyday habits that can make a huge difference in resetting your gut and feeling your best. Consistency is key — these small changes, when done daily, will build up to significant improvements over time.

Let's dive into the habits that helped me — and will help you — reset your gut and enhance your overall well-being.

1. Start Your Day with Warm Water & Lemon

I know it might sound simple, but drinking warm water with a squeeze of lemon first thing in the morning has been a game-changer for me.

Why it works:

- **Hydrates your body** after a long night of sleep, jumpstarting your digestion.
- **Lemon** helps balance pH levels and promotes bile production, aiding in detoxification.

- It **stimulates peristalsis** (the movement of your intestines), which is crucial for eliminating waste from your body.

Try sipping it slowly as soon as you wake up, and wait about 20-30 minutes before eating breakfast.

---

2. Prioritize Fiber-Rich Foods

Eating plenty of fiber-rich foods is one of the most important things you can do for your gut.

Why it works:

- **Fiber** helps regulate bowel movements by adding bulk to stool and preventing constipation.
- It feeds the **good bacteria** in your gut, promoting a healthy microbiome.
- It reduces bloating and helps regulate blood sugar levels.

Foods high in fiber include:

- **Leafy greens** (spinach, kale)
- **Whole grains** (quinoa, oats, brown rice)
- **Legumes** (lentils, chickpeas, beans)
- **Fruits** (apples, pears, berries)
- **Vegetables** (broccoli, carrots, zucchini)

---

3. Eat Mindfully and Slowly

One of the most overlooked habits is how we eat. Eating mindfully and slowly can help reduce stress on your digestive system.

Why it works:

- **Chewing thoroughly** allows your body to properly break down food, aiding digestion.

- It helps your brain register when you're full, preventing overeating.
- Eating slowly allows your gut to properly absorb nutrients, reducing bloating and discomfort.

Try setting aside time to eat without distractions like your phone or TV. Focus on the taste and texture of each bite — it'll help improve digestion and prevent overeating.

---

4. Drink Plenty of Water

Staying hydrated is essential for healthy digestion and overall well-being.

Why it works:

- **Water** helps break down food so your body can absorb nutrients more effectively.
- It softens stool and helps prevent constipation.

- It aids in detoxification and flushes out toxins from your body.

Aim to drink at least **8 glasses of water** a day. You can also incorporate herbal teas like peppermint or ginger, which are known to soothe the digestive system.

---

5. Practice Stress Management

As we've already discussed, stress is one of the biggest factors that can disrupt your gut health. So, making time each day for stress-reducing activities is crucial.

Why it works:

- Practices like **deep breathing, meditation**, or **yoga** activate your parasympathetic nervous system, allowing your body to relax and improve digestion.

- Reducing stress lowers the level of **cortisol**, the stress hormone, which can reduce inflammation in your gut.

Try starting your day with a **5-minute meditation** or end your day with a relaxing **yoga stretch**. These habits are small but powerful for long-term gut health.

---

6. Get Moving Every Day

Regular physical activity helps keep your digestive system in check.

Why it works:

- **Exercise** helps stimulate gut motility, preventing constipation.
- It increases blood flow to your digestive organs, promoting better digestion and nutrient absorption.

- It supports a healthy microbiome and balances gut bacteria.

You don't need to do intense workouts every day — even a **30-minute walk** or some gentle stretching can make a big difference in your gut health.

---

7. Get Enough Sleep

Sleep is crucial for overall health — and that includes your gut.

Why it works:

- **Quality sleep** allows your body to repair and restore itself, including your gut.
- Lack of sleep disrupts gut bacteria and impairs digestion, leading to issues like bloating, constipation, and discomfort.

- Sleep also reduces stress, which we know is important for gut health.

Aim for 7-9 hours of **quality sleep** each night. If you have trouble sleeping, try establishing a relaxing bedtime routine, such as reading or practicing mindfulness.

---

8. Incorporate Gut-Friendly Supplements

Supplements can be helpful in supporting your gut health, especially if you're dealing with digestive issues like constipation or bloating.

Probiotic Supplements: Probiotics introduce beneficial bacteria to your gut, helping balance your microbiome and support digestion.

Magnesium: Magnesium helps relax the muscles in your intestines, improving bowel movements and reducing constipation.

Digestive Enzymes: These supplements can aid in the breakdown of food and improve nutrient absorption, especially if you have trouble digesting certain foods.

Be sure to talk to a healthcare provider before starting any supplements to ensure they're right for you.

---

9. Consistency is Key

The most important thing you can do is stay consistent. Healing your gut takes time, but every small change you make builds towards long-term wellness.

Remember that no one habit will fix everything overnight. But by sticking to these simple, daily habits, you'll start to see and feel improvements in your gut health — and your overall well-being.

Conclusion

By adopting these habits, you're not just resetting your gut — you're resetting your entire body. Gut health isn't just about digestion; it's about **feeling energized, confident, and balanced**. You've taken the first step by reading this guide, and I'm so proud of you for taking charge of your health.

If you're consistent with these habits, you'll soon feel the positive changes — inside and out. Trust the process, and be kind to yourself along the way. Healing isn't a race; it's a journey.

Thank you for joining me on this gut reset journey, and I'm so excited to see how you feel after applying these changes!

www.ingramcontent.com/pod-product-compliance
Lightning Source LLC
Chambersburg PA
CBHW062143160726
48282CB00027B/931
* 9 7 8 9 3 3 4 3 0 8 1 2 9 *